Coles Notes Medical Series

THYROID PROBLEMS

A guide for patients

Ivy Fettes PhD., M.D., FRCPC.

Published by Prospero Books
2001 Toronto, Canada

© Copyright 2001 and Published by
COLES PUBLISHING. A division of Prospero Books.
Toronto – Canada

Cataloguing in Publication Data
Fettes, Ivy
Thyroid problems : a guide for patients

(Coles notes medical series)
Includes Index.
ISBN 0-7740-3868-3

I. Thyroid gland — Diseases — Popular works.   I. Title.   II Series.

RC655.F47 2000   616.4 4   C00-933114-X

Publisher: Nigel Berrisford
Medical editor: Fred Saibil, MD, FRCP(C)
Editing: Paul Kropp Communications
Cover and book design: Karen Petherick
Layout: Christine Cullen
Cover photo: Digital Imagery® copyright 1999 PhotoDisc, Inc.

Printed and bound in Canada by Webcom Limited
Cover finish: Webcom's Exclusive DURACOAT

This small book is dedicated to all people who are interested in the thyroid gland.

Special thanks go to my family and friends, especially Christopher Crerar, Dr. Joanne Lorraine and Donna Newman for their help with the manuscript.

I am also grateful to my colleagues in Medicine and Surgery who continue to teach me and inspire me and to my patients and students, who mean the world to me.

Contents

Appendices

Welcome to Coles Notes Medical Series

The information explosion of the past 20 years has been especially striking in the field of medical science. Doctors and scientists have made tremendous progress in the diagnosis and treatment of all kinds of diseases, both old and new. Coupled with this progress, there has been a dramatic change in doctor–patient relationships. Gone, for the most part, is the old "just do what I tell you, and don't ask questions" approach to treatment. Patients are now asked to take responsibility for themselves and are encouraged to participate in the decision-making process when it comes to choices of therapy.

That's why we have developed a Coles Notes medical series. Like all Coles Notes, these books are informative and concise. Written in everyday, easy-to-understand language, they should provide you with the information that you need in order to establish an effective partnership with your treatment team.

All the author-doctors involved in this project are eminent in their fields, and they all share a desire to educate the public about important medical issues. They believe that an informed patient (and family) is essential to modern medical care. An effective understanding means that you and your family have to be aware of the basic issues involved—from the diagnosis of a condition, to the ways in which the condition may progress, to the currently available management strategies. The books in the Coles Notes medical series cover all these issues. As well, these books guide you to other sources of information and support to groups across Canada. Each book has a detailed glossary at the back to explain those terms essential to your understanding.

It is our hope that these books will help you to be a better patient—or to be better equipped to support someone who is dealing with these medical issues. The treatment of a disease or condition no longer lies entirely in the hands of the physician. It requires your understanding, your consideration of treatment options, and your commitment to a treatment plan. We hope that Coles Notes will make this possible.

Fred Saibil, MD, FRCP(C)
Medical Editor, Coles Notes

Fred Saibil, MD, FRCP (C) is Head of the Division of Gastroenterology at Sunnybrook Health Science Centre as well as an Associate Professor of Medicine at the University of Toronto. He is the author of Crohn's Disease and Ulcerative Colitis *(Key Porter) and Medical Editor of the books in Coles Notes medical series.*

Introduction

The thyroid is a butterfly- or dumbbell-shaped, fleshy gland that sits in front of the windpipe, just below the larynx (sometimes called the "voice box"). The thyroid has two lobes, one on either side of the windpipe, with a thin isthmus or bridge crossing the windpipe to connect them. In an adult, the thyroid weighs about 20 grams (2/3 of an ounce).

The thyroid is a relatively small but extremely important gland that can affect the function of virtually every cell in your body. Thyroid hormones are major regulators of our growth and metabolism. Our energy production or metabolism is speeded up by an excess of thyroid hormone and slowed down by a deficiency of thyroid hormone. These conditions are called hyperthyroidism and hypothyroidism, a change of only two letters, but one that signifies very different medical problems.

Hypothyroidism, or an underactive thyroid, is the most common type of thyroid problem. In this condition everything is slowed down and you may feel tired, cold, constipated and experience an unexpected weight gain. Hypothyroidism is easily treated by replacement of the major thyroid hormone, thyroxine.

Hyperthyroidism results from too much thyroid hormone. Everything tends to be speeded up. You may feel hot, sweaty, nervous and anxious. Your heart races and you feel short of breath. You may lose weight in spite of increased appetite and thirst and eating and drinking more than usual. The choice of treatment for hyperthyroidism will depend on the cause. The possibilities include prescription medications (drugs), radioactive iodine and surgery.

Thyroid nodules may exist by themselves or in the company of other nodules in the thyroid gland. When there are several nodules in an enlarged thyroid, the condition is called a multinodular goiter. Usually there are no symptoms associated with the nodules unless they are over-producing thyroid hormone or are so large that they are causing problems with swallowing or breathing due to pressure on the esophagus or windpipe. Although thyroid nodules are almost always benign, they occasionally contain cancer cells. The treatment for thyroid cancer usually involves surgery and radioactive iodine. The response to treatment is excellent for the majority of people with thyroid cancer.

The study of the thyroid is part of endocrinology, a branch of medicine which deals with hormones, the organs that produce the hormones (often called glands) and the body tissues upon which the hormones act. Hormones are chemical messengers which may have either local or distant effects upon the body. They are produced by glands, body tissues that produce or secrete a substance. Not all glands are endocrine glands, because not all the substances secreted are hormones. For example, sweat glands release salty water as a response to exercise, heat, and stress, but they do not produce any hormones. The thyroid is an endocrine gland, and treatment of thyroid problems is often guided by an endocrinologist.

An endocrinologist is a doctor who specializes in disorders of the hormone-producing organs. Many of the clinical presentations we see in endocrinology relate to the under- or over-production of hormones. Diabetes, for instance, may be due to a deficiency of insulin, menopause to a lack of estrogen, and gigantism to an excess of growth hormone.

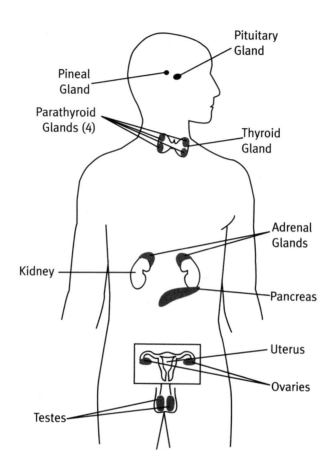

Pituitary Gland

Pineal Gland

Parathyroid Glands (4)

Thyroid Gland

Adrenal Glands

Kidney

Pancreas

Uterus

Ovaries

Testes

THE ENDOCRINE GLANDS

A Brief History of the Thyroid

nlargements of the thyroid, producing a swelling in the neck, are called goiters and have been recognized since ancient times. The Greeks apparently attributed goiters to the type of water people drank. They were at least partly correct because we know that iodine deficiency in the diet predisposes people to the development of goiters, and iodine is frequently found dissolved in water. It has been claimed that seaweed, which contains iodine, was used in treating goiters in ancient China. (The addition of iodized salt to our diets in the last 50 years has resulted in a dramatic decrease in the prevalence of goiter.)

Our understanding of the role of the thyroid gland has evolved over many thousands of years. Hippocrates (460–370 B.C.) is called the "father of medicine" and many medical students throughout the world take the "Hippocratic oath" at graduation. Hippocrates vastly expanded the art of studying the patient by urging physicians to check a person's appearance, temperature, respiration, and pulse. This facilitated our knowledge of anatomy, physiology, and internal medicine and remains a foundation in medical practice. Hippocrates is considered to have first recognized endocrinology because he described the concepts of "too much" or "too little" as a cause of disease.

It was the great physician Galen (130–200 A.D.) who described the anatomical location of the thyroid gland. Much later, Paracelsus (1493–1541) described endemic cretinism in children—a mental deficiency due to severe thyroid hormone deficiency from lack of iodine in the diet.

Thomas Wharton (1614–1673) was the first to describe the ductless glands (now called endocrine glands) and to specifically name the thyroid gland. In 1661 Neils Stensen made the clear distinction between the ductless (endocrine) glands and the lymph nodes, which are sometimes called glands, although they are not part of the endocrine glandular system.

The purpose of the thyroid gland remained unknown in the seventeenth century. Wharton thought it might be present to round out and beautify the neck. Such was the state of medicine at the time.

In the nineteenth century, Robert Graves (1796–1853) gave an excellent description of a combination of thyroid enlargement, eyeball "enlargement," and a variety of signs and symptoms that we recognize today as characteristic of an overactive thyroid gland (hyperthyroidism). Graves attributed the clinical disorder to the thyroid and henceforth the most common form of hyperthyroidism, which is due to an autoimmune disorder, is called Graves' disease.

Sir William Gull (1816–1890) was the first to describe the adult "cretinoid state" (myxedema or hypothyroidism). The disease had long been recognized in children, but he was the first to recognize it in an adult. Gull had a major interest in neurologic disease and thought that myxedema was a disorder of the nervous system. He was, of course, only partially correct.

The late nineteenth century and the twentieth century were marked by major leaps forward in our understanding of the thyroid gland. George Murray deduced that myxedema was due to lack of a particular substance in the body and decided that it was a rational approach to make up that deficiency. He first injected thyroid extract into patients in 1891 and thereby became a pioneer of thyroid replacement therapy.

The term "hormone" was first coined in about 1902 and comes from the Greek word *hormaino*, which means "to stir into action." Ernest Starling developed the concept of hormones being chemical messengers that are secreted into the bloodstream from endocrine glands.

The most common cause of hypothyroidism is recognized to be due to an autoimmune chronic thyroiditis. The condition was described by Hakaru Hashimoto in 1912 and it bears his name (Hashimoto's thyroiditis).

One of the major events to facilitate our understanding of the thyroid in the twentieth century was the development of the radioimmunoassay technique by Rosalyn Yalow and Solomon Berson in the 1960s. The ability to detect minute amounts of thyroid hormones in the blood enables doctors to detect an excess or deficiency of the hormones. These measurements have become more and more sensitive and are considered standard procedure in making the diagnosis of hyperthyroidism and hypothyroidism.

In the 1970s, a pituitary hormone called thyrotropin or thyroid stimulating hormone (TSH) and a hypothalamic hormone called thyrotropin releasing hormone (TRH) were extracted from brain tissue. This enabled scientists to begin to understand the complex interactions between the brain and the thyroid. Research has demonstrated a hierarchical system of stimulation from the hypothalamus to the pituitary and then to the thyroid, which in turn exerts negative feedback on the pituitary and hypothalamus. "Negative" feedback means that high levels turn off the stimulation and low levels turn on the stimulation. (Just like a thermostat responds to high temperatures by turning off a furnace and to low temperatures by turning it on.)

Higher Central Nervous System (Brain)
Hypothalamus

Produces TRH (Thyrotropin Releasing Hormone)
Pituitary Gland

Produces TSH (Thyroid Stimulating Hormone)
in response to TRH

Thyroid Gland
Produces T4 (Thyroxine) and some T3 (Triiodothyronine)
in response to TSH

Note 1: If too much T4 and T3 are present in the body, then TSH will be turned off (this is called negative feedback).

Note 2: If too little T4 and T3 are present in the body, then TSH will increase to try and drive the thyroid to produce more hormone.

With the rapid evolution of molecular biological techniques in the 1970s, '80s and '90s we have developed a more comprehensive knowledge base of how thyroid hormones exert their multiple and diverse effects. Worldwide there are thousands of thyroid researchers contributing to this effort. We continue to learn and develop more effective means of diagnosing and treating thyroid disease.

CHAPTER ONE

The Day-to-Day Work
of the Thyroid Gland

In order for the thyroid gland to produce the hormones that effectively regulate growth and metabolism, the gland must first synthesize or create the hormones. This is a complex process involving a number of steps.

The first step in the synthesis of thyroid hormones involves trapping iodine within the gland. The iodine comes from our diet (iodized salt is a good source) and is absorbed through the gastrointestinal system. It is then transported through the blood stream to the follicular cells of the thyroid gland.

The follicles are stimulated into activity by thyroid stimulating hormone (TSH). The cells of the follicles make a large glycoprotein (carbohydrate attached to protein) called thyroglobulin. Next, either three or four iodine molecules are bound to parts of thyroglobulin to produce the two biologically active thyroid hormones called triiodothyronine or T3 and thyroxine or T4. T3 and T4 are formed within the thyroglobulin molecule and are stored until they are released into the bloodstream to travel throughout the body.

While T4 is produced entirely from the thyroid, most (80%) of the T3 is produced by deiodination or peripheral conversion of T4 in other tissues such as the kidney, liver, heart, and pituitary. T4 can also be converted or deiodinated to an inactive substance called reverse T3 (rT3), especially in situations such as starvation or severe illness.

Conversion of T4 to T3 and Reverse T3

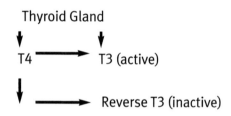

Note 1: The thyroid gland releases mostly T4 along with a small amount of T3.

Note 2: Most T3 (80%) comes from the conversion of T4 to T3 outside the thyroid gland.

Note 3: T4 is also converted to reverse T3, which is inactive, in unusual situations such as severe illness or starvation.

Thyroid hormones are essential for normal development and for maintenance of metabolic stability. Thyroid hormones affect the metabolism of carbohydrates, protein, fat, vitamins, minerals, and other hormones.

Thyroid hormone stimulates thermogenesis
or heat production. Excess levels of thyroid hormone,
as in hyperthyroidism, are associated
with the sensation of feeling hot. Deficiencies
are associated with feeling cold.

There are important interactions between thyroid
hormones and noradrenaline (norepinephrine), with an
increase in the production of norepinephrine in
hyperthyroidism and a decrease in hypothyroidism. The
hyperthyroid person feels "speeded up," and
the hypothyroid person feels "slowed down."

T4 and T3 in the blood are largely bound (attached) to plasma proteins, mostly thyroxine binding globulin (TBG). It is, however, the free or unbound fraction that determines the metabolic activity. TBG can be increased by pregnancy, oral contraceptives and some drugs such as phenothiazines. TBG can be decreased by severe malnutrition, severe illness, nephrotic syndrome, and some drugs such as anabolic steroids or phenytoin. Although changes in TBG will affect total thyroid hormone levels, they will not affect free hormone levels. Measurement of total thyroid hormone concentrations includes both protein-bound and free hormone. The measurement of free thyroid hormone concentrations are more reflective of the true thyroid status.

Thyroid hormone levels are maintained within narrow limits by a regulatory mechanism that involves the brain. Their production is regulated by a pituitary hormone called thyroid stimulating hormone (TSH). The production of TSH is, in turn, regulated by a hypothalamic hormone called thyrotropin releasing hormone (TRH). Brain centers higher than the pituitary and hypothalamus can also affect hypothalamic functions. Thus there is an axis or hierarchy of regulation. (See the diagram of axis on page xxi.)

The thyroid can exert negative feedback (see diagram on page 5) on the pituitary and hypothalamus, with low levels of T4 and T3 stimulating TSH secretion and high levels of T4 and T3 suppressing TSH secretion. The regulatory mechanism is very sensitive to small changes in circulating hormone levels. When there are low levels of T4 and T3 due to decreased activity of the thyroid gland, the level of TSH will be elevated. Thus, in hypothyroidism due to primary thyroid disease, the levels of the thyroid hormones will be reduced and the levels of TSH increased. If, however, there is pituitary or hypothalamic disease (a rare condition), the TSH will also be low. In this case the thyroid hormone levels will be low because of a failure of the pituitary to stimulate the thyroid gland. This accounts for less than 2% of the causes of hypothyroidism and is known as secondary hypothyroidism. More than 98% of people with hypothyroidism have hypothyroidism due to thyroid failure—called primary hypothyroidism.

Hyperthyroidism due to primary thyroid disease is associated with high levels of T4 and T3 and low levels of

TSH. The high circulating levels of the thyroid hormones "turn off" the production of TSH. Very rarely, hyperthyroidism is due to overproduction of TSH from a benign pituitary tumor. In this scenario all the levels—TSH, T4, and T3—will be elevated.

Feedback Systems for Thyroid Hormones

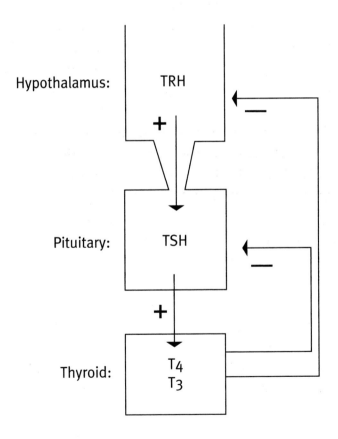

Table of Primary and Secondary Causes of Hypothyroidism

Primary hypothyroidism refers to problems affecting the thyroid gland itself. In secondary hypothyroidism, the thyroid is normal and the problem is outside the gland.

Causes of Primary Hypothyroidism	Causes of Secondary Hypothyroidism
Thyroid inflammation or infection (examples: chronic autoimmune thyroiditis, viral thyroiditis)	Hypothalamic problems (tumors, radiation, trauma, infiltration of the gland, surgery, ischemia = damage due to decreased blood supply)
Radiation (examples: therapeutic radioactive iodine or head and neck radiation for cancer)	Pituitary gland problems (same list as for hypothalamus)
Thyroid surgery	Resistance to the action of thyroid hormones
Iodine deficiency	
Other (including some medications, infiltrative diseases and congenital defects)	

Table of Primary and Secondary Causes of Hyperthyroidism

Primary hyperthyroidism refers to an overactive thyroid due to a problem in the thyroid gland itself. Secondary refers to problems originating outside the thyroid that secondarily cause an elevation in thyroid hormone levels.

Causes of Primary Hyperthyroidism	Causes of Secondary Hyperthyroidism
Inflammatory diseases (examples: Graves' disease, subacute thyroiditis, silent thyroiditis)	Excess use of thyroid medication TSH produced in excess by the pituitary gland (rare)
Thyroid nodule(s) producing too much thyroid hormone (most commonly benign nodules; rarely cancer)	Excess stimulation of thyroid gland by factors with TSH-like properties (example: hCG)
	Other, including iodine, drug side effects and more rarely ovarian tumors

The most common cause of both hypothyroidism and hyperthyroidism is autoimmune disease. "Autoimmune" literally means "immune to self." In this kind of disease, the body begins to produce antibodies that attack a particular cell, tissue, or organ. Why these autoantibodies develop is unknown, but the effects may be serious.

The hyperthyroidism of Graves' disease is due to autoantibodies that stimulate thyroid hormone production. The autoantibodies are proteins known as IgG immunoglobulins, which act like TSH and bind to and activate the thyroid follicular cells. For this reason, they are called thyroid stimulating antibodies (TSab) and can be measured in the blood. The TSab stimulate thyroid growth as well as thyroid function and may produce thyroid enlargement.

In areas like North America, where there is sufficient iodine in the diet, the most common cause of hypothyroidism is chronic autoimmune disease of the thyroid (Hashimoto's disease). In this case, the thyroid antibodies are not believed to cause the disease but rather to be associated with it. Higher levels of thyroid antibodies may indicate more advanced disease and may influence when treatment is started. Chronic autoimmune thyroiditis tends to cause a progressive and persistent failure of the thyroid gland.

Autoimmune thyroid disease is much more common in women, and it tends to run in families. Occasionally it may be associated with other autoimmune diseases such as diabetes mellitus (type 1 diabetes), gonadal failure, malabsorption syndromes, and pernicious anemia.

In remote areas of severe iodine deficiency, virtually everyone has a goiter; this is called endemic goiter. This may result in primary hypothyroidism with high levels of TSH. If there are inadequate levels of thyroid hormone during fetal life, there may be permanent neurologic damage. Cretins are the most severe example. There are also combinations of hypothyroidism and a variety of neurologic defects including mental retardation, deafness, mutism, dwarfism and spastic dysplegia. Cretinism can be prevented with the addition of iodine to the diet. If the mother's diet contains enough iodine, then the fetus will receive enough iodine. In areas of endemic goiter, the addition of iodine is more effective in preventing the goiter than reducing the size of an already existing goiter.

Both extremes of iodine intake—deficiency and excess—can result in hypothyroidism. Conversely, the administration of iodine may actually cause hyperthyroidism, particularly in people with pre-existing thyroid diseases such as autonomously functioning thyroid nodules. Only minute amounts of iodine are required for normal production of thyroid hormones. The recommended daily intake for adults is about 150 micrograms with an increase to 200 micrograms during pregnancy. One teaspoon of table salt contains 420 micrograms of iodine, which is far more iodine than we need in a day. A pinch of salt contains about 50 micrograms of iodine, as does an 8 ounce glass of milk. In Western nations, there is no need to take iodine supplements (e.g., seaweed or kelp).

Thyroid Function Tests

Most Sensitive Thyroid Function Tests

TSH

free T4

free T3

The most sensitive blood tests for assessment of thyroid function are TSH, free T4 and free T3. The levels of free T4 and free T3 measure the thyroid hormones that are not bound to proteins and are readily available to the tissues.

With primary thyroid disease, abnormalities in TSH will be seen even before abnormalities in free T4 or free T3. TSH is the most sensitive indicator of early thyroid dysfunction. Small changes in free T4 result in much larger changes in the TSH level.

The TSH level is used to detect underactivity and overactivity of the thyroid gland. TSH is used in screening all newborns for congenital hypothyroidism. It is also used for screening high-risk groups such as the elderly and individuals with suggestive symptoms who may be predisposed due to a strong family history of thyroid disease, individuals with a personal history of autoimmune disease, or women who have recently delivered a baby.

TSH is also used to monitor the dose of thyroid

"replacement" therapy for people with hypothyroidism and the dose of thyroid "suppressive" therapy for people with thyroid nodules or thyroid cancer. Typically the goal is that TSH is normalized for replacement therapy and deliberately suppressed below normal levels to prevent tumor growth.

Measurement of thyroid antibodies can provide evidence for autoimmune disease affecting the thyroid gland. In Hashimoto's disease the levels of antimicrosomal antibodies and thyroglobulin antibodies will be elevated. In Graves' disease, there is an elevation of thyroid stimulating antibodies.

Levels of the protein thyroglobulin are used in the follow-up of people with thyroid cancer who have had a thyroidectomy (complete removal of the thyroid) or destruction with radioactive iodine. Since thyroglobulin is an indicator of functioning thyroid tissue, it can be used as a "tumor marker" for evidence of recurrence of the cancer. It should be absent from the blood after complete removal of the thyroid; if it isn't, or if the level increases, then this is a sign that cancer may be present.

TRH stimulation tests, in which TRH is injected and the levels of TSH are monitored over the next one to two hours, are mostly used to assess pituitary function. For patients suffering pituitary failure, TSH levels are low and do not respond to TRH. This is unlike primary thyroid failure where the TSH levels are elevated and show an exaggerated increase with administration of TRH.

Thyroid Imaging Studies

> **Imaging the Thyroid**
>
> Ultrasound
>
> Radioisotope Scans
>
> CT Scan
>
> Magnetic Resonance Imaging

Ultrasound of the thyroid is helpful in evaluating thyroid nodules (lumps). The ultrasound provides a more accurate determination of the size of a nodule than a doctor's palpation (feeling) of the gland. Sometimes the physician can feel only one nodule but on ultrasound there are several (i.e., the gland is multinodular). The size of the nodules can be monitored over time with an ultrasound. An increase in size often leads to further testing.

Ultrasound is helpful in the distinction between cystic lesions, which are typically benign and solid lesions which are usually benign but may be malignant. Ultrasound is also used in guiding a needle biopsy (fine needle aspiration) of a nodule, particularly if the nodule is small.

Nuclear medicine techniques for imaging the thyroid include the use of iodine or technetium. The uptake of a small amount of radioactive iodine (I131 or I123) is used in distinguishing different causes of hyperthyroidism. When there is an acute inflammation of the thyroid gland, the uptake of iodine is decreased. With Graves' disease there is an increase in uptake. In Graves' disease we use the measured uptake to help calculate the dose of radioactive iodine that will be used to treat the disease. With higher uptakes, lower doses of I131 can be used for partial or total destruction of the overactive tissue. When hyperthyroidism is due to overactivity of one or more thyroid nodules ("toxic nodules"), the uptake of iodine will be concentrated in these "hot" nodules.

Technetium, like iodine, can be trapped by the thyroid gland. It cannot, however, be used by the body to produce thyroid hormone. Technetium scans of the thyroid can distinguish between functioning ("warm" or "hot") and non-functioning ("cold") tissue. A cold nodule is much more likely to be malignant than is a warm or hot nodule. In Graves' disease there will be an even or homogeneous uptake of technetium on the thyroid scan. If toxic nodules are present, the technetium will be concentrated in the nodules.

Computerized tomography (CT) or magnetic resonance imaging (MR or MRI) are two other scanning techniques that may be used by your doctor. They can identify metastatic lesions of thyroid cancer, including any spread of the disease to the lymph nodes. These scans may also be used to assess a goiter that is substernal (that is, extending behind the breastbone), or to monitor the appearance of thyroid tissue that remains after thyroid surgery.

CHAPTER TWO

The Underactive Thyroid (Hypothyroidism)

hyroid gland failure results in a deficiency of thyroid hormone. It affects at least 2% of the population and as many as 15% of high-risk groups, such as people over the age of 75. At the other end of the age spectrum, one in every four thousand babies in North America is born with an underactive thyroid. Statistically, an underactive thyroid is more common in females and is more common with advancing age.

Manifestations

Signs of Hypothyroidism

Fatigue

Feeling cold

Weight gain

Constipation

There are many signs and symptoms of thyroid hormone deficiency because so many organ systems can be affected. In general, everything is "slowed down," but different individuals can show different manifestations of the condition.

- Children with hypothyroidism may have reduced growth and development, both mentally and physically.
- In children and adults there may be lethargy and fatigue. You may be depressed. There is a decrease in memory and mental agility. Hearing may be impaired and speech may be slower. Movements also seem to slow down. There is a decrease is muscle tone and you may have muscle weakness. Puffiness or swelling of the face, hands, and feet may occur. Your scalp hair may be coarse and dry, and your skin may be dry and scaly. Your voice may deepen and become somewhat hoarse.
- People with hypothyroidism often complain of feeling cold (cold intolerance), being constipated, and gaining weight in spite of eating the same amount of food.
- Hypothyroidism can cause menstrual irregularities in women and infertility in both women and men. Usually women with hypothyroidism have heavier periods, but if the condition is not treated the periods may stop altogether (amenorrhea).
- With hypothyroidism, the heart rate and therefore the pulse may be slower and the blood pressure may be mildly elevated.

Although the incidence of hypothyroidism increases with age, the diagnosis may be missed because so many of the symptoms are similar to those of aging itself. Features that may suggest an underactive thyroid include depression, slow movement, constipation, dry skin, and puffiness ("water bags") under the eyes. With more severe hypothyroidism, there may be increased chance of heart failure.

Causes

Causes of Hypothyroidism

Hashimoto's thyroiditis

After treatment for an overactive thyroid

Transient inflammation

External radiation to the neck

Other

The most common cause of hypothyroidism is chronic autoimmune thyroiditis (Hashimoto's thyroiditis). There are variants of Hashimoto's thyroiditis in which the thyroid enlarges in adolescent females (juvenile thyroiditis), or becomes smaller (atrophic thyroiditis), which is usually later in life. At 4 to 12 months after delivery of a baby, the mother may experience a transient inflammation of the thyroid gland, called postpartum thyroiditis. This is manifest initially as hyperthyroidism, to be followed by hypothyroidism, and then finally a return to normal function. Postpartum thyroiditis is thought to be a variant of autoimmune thyroiditis.

The second most common cause of hypothyroidism in North America is that related to the treatment of an overactive thyroid. Treatments that may result in an underactive thyroid include radioactive iodine therapy, which may destroy the gland, and thyroid surgery.

External radiation to the neck for head and neck cancer can cause hypothyroidism. The diagnosis may not be suspected because any fatigue or weakness may be attributed to the effects of the cancer itself. Some cancers (e.g., lymphomas) may invade the thyroid gland directly. The thyroid gland may also be infiltrated by abnormal proteins or inflammatory material, as in the conditions amyloidosis and sarcoidosis, both of which are non-malignant conditions.

There are antithyroid drugs, which are used specifically to decrease thyroid hormone production in people who suffer from hyperthyroidism. Other drugs may also cause hypothyroidism, including lithium (used to control mood disorders) and amiodarone (used to control irregularities of the heart rhythm). They can block the release of thyroid hormone, but usually only in people who have a susceptibility to thyroid disease.

Sometimes the thyroid gland can become inflamed in a condition called subacute thyroiditis. In the majority of such cases, this is preceded by a viral infection involving the upper respiratory tract. The thyroid enlarges somewhat, and is tender to touch. You may have neck pain, often going up to the throat, jaws, and ears. The pain and tenderness may shift from one side (lobe) of the thyroid to the other during this illness. The cells of the thyroid gland, when inflamed, become damaged and release excessive amounts of thyroid hormones, causing symptoms of hyperthyroidism. The symptoms of overactive thyroid may last for four to six weeks and may then be followed by a transient (two to eight week) period of hypothyroidism. The symptoms of this hypothyroidism are usually mild and do not require treatment. Your thyroid function ultimately returns to normal.

Deficiencies of pituitary TSH or hypothalamic TRH account for less than 2% of cases of hypothyroidism. TSH deficiency may be due to destruction of the pituitary cells that secrete TSH. This is usually caused by a pituitary tumor, or may result from surgery or radiation therapy used to treat such a tumor. Occasionally there may be necrosis (tissue breakdown) of the pituitary after a severe post-partum bleed. Tumors other than pituitary tumors (e.g., craniopharyngioma, metastatic cancers), or infiltrative diseases (e.g., tuberculosis, hemochromatosis, histoplasmosis) may cause deficiencies of TSH and TRH. Radiation therapy to the head for malignancies may also cause a TRH deficiency. It should be noted that when TRH is deficient, TSH will also be low because there will be no stimulus message from above for the pituitary gland to produce TSH.

Generalized resistance to thyroid hormones is a rare hereditary disorder that may be mistaken for hypothyroidism or hyperthyroidism. The thyroid is enlarged, and there are elevations in free T4 and free T3 and possibly mild elevations in TSH. A number of gene mutations have been identified in this syndrome.

Although iodine deficiency is the most common cause of hypothyroidism in the world, it represents an extremely rare cause in North America, which is an "iodine-rich" area. Other rare causes of hypothyroidism are congenital defects in the thyroid's ability to produce thyroid hormone.

Laboratory Testing In Hypothyroidism

> **Lab Tests for Primary Hypothyroidism**
>
> TSH
>
> Free T4 if TSH elevated
>
> Thyroid antibodies

TSH is the single best blood test to evaluate thyroid function when we suspect primary hypothyroidism. In early hypothyroidism, the TSH will be elevated before the free T4 drops below normal. As the thyroid failure advances, both tests will be abnormal, with a high TSH and a low free T4 level.

When hypothyroidism is due to pituitary or hypothalamic disease (secondary hypothyroidism), TSH levels will be normal or low. In such cases, the thyroid status is best assessed by the level of free T4, which will be low in hypothyroidism.

Blood levels of antibodies to a substance named thyroid microsomal antigen (thyroid peroxidase) are measured to confirm a suspected diagnosis of autoimmune chronic thyroiditis.

Case History A

A 75-year-old woman presents to her doctor's office in July. She is wearing her winter coat. She is accompanied by her daughter, who describes her mother as having slowed down in the past few months. She has also noted puffy bags under her mother's eyes. The patient herself feels exhausted and lethargic, and has been off her usually excellent bridge game. She feels that her speech and movements are slower than usual. She has been wearing her winter sweaters around her house, despite the very warm humid weather outside. She reluctantly admits to using quite a bit of laxative for some troublesome constipation. Despite sleeping at least 10 hours a night, the patient needs to take a nap in the afternoon as well, which is quite unusual for her. The patient herself looks quite sad, and the daughter is concerned that her mother might be depressed.

Comments

This 75-year-old woman has many of the symptoms of hypothyroidism. A screening TSH should be ordered in elderly women presenting with these complaints. If indeed the TSH is high, suggesting an underactive thyroid, then replacement therapy with L-thyroxine will make a considerable improvement in this woman's life. Many if not all of her symptoms may resolve completely once her thyroid hormone levels are back to normal. When initiating replacement therapy in a person of this age, the general rule is to start with low doses and increase the dose gradually until the TSH has normalized.

Case History B

A 60-year-old man who had cancer of the vocal cords (larynx) was treated with neck surgery and radiation 5 years ago. He is feeling weak and tired and no longer able to walk his golden retriever, who used to enjoy long outings twice a day. Strangely enough, the dog also seems to be very tired and is just sleeping all day. Both the patient and his dog have gained some weight.

Comments

Both the patient and his dog may have underactive thyroid conditions—in both species an underactive thyroid is the most common thyroid problem! In the case of the patient, his thyroid may have been damaged by the radiation given previously for his vocal cord cancer, leading to loss of thyroid hormone production. Replacement of thyroid hormone for both man and dog should lead to a resumption of their pleasurable outdoor adventures.

Case History C

A 50-year-old highly successful business woman presents to her doctor feeling somewhat slowed down and depressed (in other words, unable to keep up with her usual 12-hour-a-day work schedule)! She wonders if she, like her mother, might have an underactive thyroid. Her mother has been on thyroid hormone replacement therapy for more than 20 years. Blood tests in this patient confirm a high TSH and the presence of thyroid antibodies.

Comments

Thyroid disease is more common in women than in men and tends to run in families. The high TSH in her blood test confirms an underactive thyroid. The thyroid antibodies indicate that the cause is Hashimoto's thyroiditis, a chronic autoimmune disease of the thyroid gland. This patient, like her mother, will require long-term thyroid hormone replacement therapy.

Case History D

A 30-year-old woman delivered her first baby six months ago. The delivery was successful, and the baby healthy, but the patient finds herself inexplicably depressed and completely worn out. She is having trouble looking after her beautiful new baby, and is feeling very guilty about this. Her mother-in-law has been making some unhelpful comments about her lack of skills as a mother. Her husband is supportive and concerned, and he has come to the doctor's appointment with his wife.

Comments

This woman may have a condition called postpartum thyroiditis or she may be suffering from postpartum depression. Her doctor will order a TSH level to determine which is the most accurate diagnosis. In this case, it is postpartum thyroiditis, an inflammatory condition of the thyroid that occurs within three to eight months after delivery. Patients most commonly present with an overactive thyroid, but some patients such as this woman present in the underactive phase of this condition. If the underactivity of the thyroid is severe, then temporary replacement with thyroid hormone may be needed. Most patients do not require thyroid hormone, and can be reassured that their symptoms will resolve spontaneously within weeks to a few months. Postpartum thyroiditis may recur with subsequent pregnancies, and may indicate an increased risk for other thyroid problems in the future.

Case History E

A 25-year-old woman received 8 millicuries of radioactive iodine as treatment for Graves' hyperthyroidism one year ago. She is now complaining that her arms and legs are feeling heavy. She is gaining weight and is constipated. Her menstrual periods have become heavier and longer, lasting seven days instead of her usual five days. Her skin and hair are dry.

Comments

This woman received appropriate treatment for an overactive thyroid due to Graves' disease. However, one of the risks of radioactive iodine therapy is the development of an underactive thyroid, as can be seen in this woman. People who have received radioactive iodine should be monitored with respect to their thyroid function. Usually the TSH level will start to rise before a patient develops any symptoms, and replacement therapy can be initiated before the symptoms become severe. All this patient's symptoms will go away when she is on adequate thyroid hormone replacement therapy. Because she is young, and generally healthy, this patient can be started on her full estimated replacement dose right away.

Treatment

When a diagnosis of chronic or permanent hypothyroidism has been made, lifelong thyroid hormone replacement is required. The treatment of hypothyroidism is with L-thyroxine (T4), which is a standardized and inexpensive medication.

The usual replacement dose of L-thyroxine is 1.7 micrograms of drug per kg of body weight per day. However, the dose required may vary from 0.05 milligrams (50 micrograms) to 1.5 milligrams (150 micrograms) per day or more, depending on your weight, age, and the degree of thyroid failure. In elderly people, or those with known heart disease such as angina, we start at a very low dose, such as 0.025 milligrams (25 micrograms) per day and then gradually increase. Thyroid hormone is taken with water first thing in the morning. It is better absorbed when taken on an empty stomach, without food or vitamins or other medications.

The dosage of thyroid hormone is gradually adjusted (usually every four to six weeks) until there is normalization of the TSH level. Most signs and symptoms of hypothyroidism disappear in one to two months, although some abnormalities may persist for four to six months.

Once your TSH is normalized, periodic follow-up of the TSH level and assessment for the signs and symptoms of hypothyroidism are done every six to twelve months. In pregnancy the TSH levels are followed more often, as the dose of thyroid hormone may have to be increased during pregnancy.

Transient hypothyroidism, as in subacute thyroiditis or postpartum thyroiditis, may not require replacement with thyroid hormone. In medication-induced hypothyroidism, such as that due to lithium or amiodarone, consideration should be given to stopping the offending drug. This may not always be possible, depending on the reason for the drug.

CHAPTER THREE

The Overactive Thyroid (Hyperthyroidism)

Manifestations

Many of the symptoms and signs of hyperthyroidism or "thyrotoxicosis" reflect a speeding up or acceleration of body functions.

Feeling nervous, anxious, hot, and sweaty are common manifestations. People around you may complain to you about your edginess and irritability.

Signs of Hyperthyroidism

Nervousness

Feeling hot

Racing heart

Weight loss

You may have a sensation that your heart is racing and it is! In spite of an increase in appetite, most people with hyperthyroidism lose weight. You may notice an increase in the number of daily bowel movements; if you were constipated before, you may find that your bowel movements have become more regular.

You may be experiencing a decrease in the ability to do exercises and sports because of shortness of breath, weakness and tiring easily. People with hyperthyroidism sometimes look "startled"; your eyes may be more prominent. The thyroid gland is usually enlarged and may be visible in the neck.

People may notice that you are talking and moving more quickly than usual. As the saying goes, you'll "talk a mile a minute." You will find it difficult to sit quietly. Your hands are likely to be shaky or tremulous and feel warm and moist. This is unlike people who are anxious, but not hyperthyroid, who may have sweaty palms that are cool to the touch.

Elderly people with hyperthyroidism may be "apathetic" (showing lack of interest in anything), unlike their younger counterparts who are "hyper" in activity and behavior. The most common manifestations of hyperthyroidism in an older person are weight loss and heart problems, including a rapid irregular heart rate and pulse and shortness of breath due to heart failure.

There is usually no neck pain or tenderness associated with an overactive thyroid, unless the hyperthyroidism is due to inflammation of the thyroid gland as in subacute thyroiditis.

Some manifestations of hyperthyroidism are only

found in Graves' disease. These include enlargement of the eye muscles, which may cause a bulging forward of the eyes and may interfere with normal eye movements and vision. Two other findings that are more rare are patches of abnormal (leathery and hard) skin over the shins and thickening of the tissue at the base of the fingernails, leading to a bulb-like appearance of the fingertips (called "clubbing").

Causes

Causes of Hyperthyroidism

Graves' disease

Toxic or "hot" nodule(s)

Subacute thyroiditis

Silent thyroiditis

Other

Hyperthyroidism occurs in about 2% of women in North America. It is much less common in men and in children.

By far the most common cause of hyperthyroidism is Graves' disease, which is an autoimmune disease associated with the presence of thyroid-stimulating antibodies. Graves' disease can occur in children and adults of any age, but is most common in women between the ages of

30 and 60. Typically there are multiple symptoms of hyperthyroidism. The thyroid is diffusely (evenly) enlarged and very actively takes up iodine for the production of thyroid hormone. The overproduction of thyroid hormone turns off TSH and so TSH levels are very low. Although people with hyperthyroidism of any cause may appear to have a "stare," it is only in Graves' disease that there may be enlargement and abnormal function of the eye muscles (the medical term for this is ophthalmopathy).

Hyperthyroidism may develop in people, usually women over 60, who have had a multinodular goiter for years, in fact, decades. The number of nodules is variable. As the nodules grow, they can become overactive, with an increase in the production of the thyroid hormones T4 and T3. Sometimes single (solitary) nodules are the cause of hyperthyroidism. Nodules that oversecrete (overproduce) thyroid hormone are called "toxic" or "hot" nodules because the nodules show an increase in the uptake of radioactive iodine (or technetium) when scanned.

The next most common cause of hyperthyroidism is thyroid inflammation, which may be painful, as in subacute thyroiditis, or painless, as in silent thyroiditis. Subacute thyroiditis usually follows a viral respiratory infection. Like Graves' disease, silent thyroiditis is thought to be autoimmune in nature. However, unlike Graves' disease, silent thyroiditis occurs in nearly equal numbers of men and women. Women who have recently delivered a baby appear to be particularly predisposed to silent thyroiditis.

With both silent and subacute thyroiditis, there is an

acute or sudden release of thyroid hormone due to inflammation of the gland, with disruption of the thyroid follicular cells. The effects are short-lived and the symptoms of hyperthyroidism will usually disappear within six weeks. Because of the disruption of the thyroid cells, the gland is unable to take up iodine from the blood, and the hyperthyroid phase is usually followed by a hypothyroid phase before the gland recovers and returns to normal function.

If you are on thyroid hormone as replacement therapy (treatment) for hypothyroidism but are taking more than the body needs, you may have signs and symptoms of hyperthyroidism.

Some drugs that contain iodine (e.g., amiodarone) may precipitate hyperthyroidism. This is usually found in people with a pre-existing thyroid abnormality such as Graves' disease or nodular goiter.

A rare cause of hyperthyroidism is a pituitary tumor. Such a tumor produces excessive amounts of TSH, which, in turn, overstimulates the thyroid gland. Unlike other causes of hyperthyroidism, where the TSH level is low, the TSH level in these people is very high. The levels of the thyroid hormones are also high.

Causes of hyperthyroidism that are even more rare are those due to thyroid tissue found in abnormal locations in the body (such as the ovary), thyroid cancer, and to tumors that overproduce a hormone called hCG (human chorionic gonadotropin), which acts a bit like TSH. Thyroid hormone resistance, a rare condition that often runs in families, may be confused with hyperthyroidism because of high levels of thyroid hormone found on a blood test. Although most people with this condition have an enlarged thyroid gland (goiter), they do not have symptoms of an overactive thyroid. Thyroid hormone resistance should be diagnosed and managed by an endocrinologist.

Laboratory Testing

TSH is the appropriate screening test for hyperthyroidism, just as it is for hypothyroidism. TSH levels in the blood will be low in all causes of hyperthyroidism except for TSH-producing pituitary tumors and thyroid hormone resistance.

The next step is measurement of free T4 and free T3. In hyperthyroidism due to Graves' disease or toxic nodules, the free T3 is usually elevated out of proportion to the free T4. Usually both levels are high. A small percentage of people with toxic nodules will have a high T3 but normal T4, and this is called "T3 toxicosis." An elevation in free T3 may be the first sign of recurrent hyperthyroidism in patients who have been treated for Graves' disease. In hyperthyroidism due to inflammatory conditions such as subacute or viral thyroiditis, there is more likely to be an elevation in free T4 without an elevation in free T3.

In the majority of people with hyperthyroidism, the TSH will be low and the free T4 will be high. The exceptions are people with TSH secreting pituitary tumors and thyroid hormone resistance, in which TSH and free T4 will both be elevated.

In hyperthyroidism due to Graves' disease, the whole gland is overactive or hyperfunctioning. This condition can be assessed by measurement of the uptake of radioactive iodine in the gland; it will be high. Although people with subacute or viral thyroiditis may be hyperthyroid, this is due to the excessive release of already-formed hormone rather than to overproduction of hormone. The thyroid cells in these two conditions are temporarily disrupted, and cannot take up radioactive iodine, and thus the measured uptake will be low.

Thyroid scans with radioisotopes such as technetium or radioactive iodine are also used to identify one or more toxic or "hot" nodules. The uptake is increased in the region of the toxic nodule and decreased in the rest of the gland.

Measurement of thyroid-stimulating antibodies (TSab, also called thyroid-stimulating immunoglobulin or TS Ig) may be done to confirm a diagnosis of Graves' disease. It may also be used to assess the response to treatment and to predict the recurrence of the disease. High TSab levels in a pregnant woman can forecast the development of Graves' disease in her newborn baby.

Case History A

A 31-year-old woman is complaining of nervousness, difficulty concentrating, a racing pulse, and scanty menstrual periods. She has lost 10 pounds without trying. She feels as if there is a lump in her throat. Her friends and co-workers have found her quite jumpy and are urging her to seek help.

Comments

This woman may well have an overactive thyroid due to Graves' disease. The initial investigations to confirm an overactive thyroid would be blood tests to check for a low TSH level and elevated thyroid hormone level (free T4 and sometimes free T3 levels). If the diagnosis of an overactive thyroid is confirmed by blood tests, a radioactive uptake scan is still required to determine the exact cause of the overactivity. (Is there one hot nodule? Are there multiple hot nodules? Is the whole gland generally "hot" on nuclear tracer uptake or is the gland cold, suggesting a different diagnosis...?) In Graves' disease, the whole gland will be "hot," indicating a diffuse overactivity of the thyroid. Once the diagnosis of Graves' disease is confirmed, treatment must commence because the patient's symptoms could worsen considerably without therapy. The treatment will likely include both a beta-blocking drug to slow her racing heart and an additional drug to decrease thyroid hormone production.

Case History B

A 70-year-old woman, who has had a nodular (lumpy) goiter for about 40 years, has noticed the recent development of shakiness in both her hands, and a rapid fluttering in her heart. She has lost 20 pounds and is worried that she might have cancer. Ironically, her cat also appears to be anxious and agitated and is losing weight in spite of eating constantly.

Comments

Both the patient and her cat may have overactive thyroid conditions due to "toxic" or "hot" nodules in the thyroid gland. It is not unusual to develop one or more hot nodules in an enlarged thyroid gland that contains multiple nodules. In older people, the symptoms of an overactive thyroid often include a fine shaking of the hands, a rapid irregular heart beat, or even apathy. This patient probably has atrial fibrillation as a cause of her fluttering heart.

Making a diagnosis in this patient will once again involve blood testing for TSH and thyroid hormone levels, and a nuclear medicine scan to look for "hot" nodules. The treatment for a "hot" multinodular goiter in a 70-year-old person will include a beta blocker and an antithyroid drug to "cool" her down, followed by definitive therapy with radioactive iodine. Interestingly, the cat will also require treatment! Fortunately, both the patient and her pet have an excellent prognosis—at least in terms of their thyroid conditions.

Case History C

An 83-year-old woman has become withdrawn and depressed. Her family feel that she is "wasting away." Her clothes, which once fit somewhat snugly, are now just hanging on her. The patient and her family are concerned about the possibility of cancer.

Comments

An overactive thyroid in an older person may in fact present as apathy, weight loss, and depression—but these symptoms may well have other causes. Depression itself is common in the elderly and may cause loss of appetite and significant weight loss. A screening TSH level will be required in this patient as in other patients in whom thyroid disease is suspected. An underlying cancer is certainly possible and should be considered and investigated if the TSH comes back normal. The most likely cause of hyperthyroidism in this patient would be Graves' disease.

Case History D

A 23-year-old student, who is about to go back to college, is complaining of pain in his neck. He was working outdoors for the summer and at the end of the summer had a bad cold and sore throat. Now he has pain and tenderness on the outside of the neck, and there is some fullness in his neck just under his Adam's apple. He is feeling hot and his pulse has increased from his usual 60 beats per minute to 90 beats per minute.

Comments

This is a classic history for a patient with subacute thyroiditis—a painful inflammatory condition of the thyroid gland that nearly always is preceded by a viral upper respiratory infection. Most head colds are *not* followed by subacute thyroiditis, but most subacute thyroiditis is preceded by a viral type head cold or chest infection. The usual screening blood tests of TSH and thyroid hormone levels should be ordered, as well as additional blood tests such as the erythrocyte sedimentation rate (ESR). The ESR is a nonspecific measure of inflammation and can be used to follow the illness. A radioactive iodine uptake in this case will be low. (Due to the inflammation in the gland, iodine cannot be trapped and taken up by the thyroid gland.)

Treatment involves aspirin-type compounds for pain relief, and very rarely corticosteroids such as prednisone, for an additional anti-inflammatory effect. Beta blockers may be used transiently to control heart rate. This student would be expected to make a full recovery within weeks, although he may experience a brief phase of underactive thyroid activity before finally returning to normal thyroid function (overactive ➠ underactive ➠ recovery).

Case History E

A 55-year-old woman has been on the same dose of thyroid replacement for 25 years, following the original diagnosis of underactive thyroid. She is having trouble sleeping at night and can feel her heart pounding in her chest.

Comments

It is very common for a person to have varying thyroid hormone replacement needs over time. TSH should be checked in this woman to make certain she is not taking more replacement than she currently needs. If the TSH is indeed low, suggesting over-replacement, then her thyroid hormone dose should be slowly tapered until the TSH is in the normal range. Her sleep will likely improve and the palpitations resolve as her thyroid hormone levels return to the normal range. The patient may feel subjectively more tired as her dose is lowered, even though her thyroid hormone testing is normalizing. In the long run, this patient will feel better and there will be less risk to her heart from a chronic rapid heart rate. Over-replacement with thyroid hormones can increase the risk of osteoporosis (bone loss) in women lacking in estrogen, and it would be important to prevent this as well.

Treatment

The treatment of hyperthyroidism will depend on the cause and on the severity of the symptoms. For people with mild and transient symptoms, as in silent thyroiditis or subacute thyroiditis, no treatment may be needed.

Drugs such as beta-adrenergic blockers, commonly known as "beta blockers" (e.g., propranolol), which decrease the effects of high circulating levels of thyroid hormone, can be used in hyperthyroidism from any cause. These medications slow your pulse and decrease the nervousness, tremor, and heat intolerance. You will feel more comfortable within days. These drugs do not decrease the production of thyroid hormone from the thyroid gland. Fortunately, they will not interfere with the routine laboratory testing that may be required to make the correct diagnosis.

Treatment for Graves' Disease

In Graves' hyperthyroidism, beta blockers alone will not be enough to treat the disease. The two best treatments for Graves' disease are radioactive iodine (I131) and antithyroid drugs.

In many cases, a small dose (6 to 12 millicuries) of radioactive iodine may be given as a single capsule as the treatment for hyperthyroidism due to Graves' disease. The capsule is simply swallowed, with water, in an outpatient setting. This radiation has no effects on the rest of your body. This treatment reduces the amount of functioning thyroid tissue over the next weeks, months, and years.

There is usually restoration of normal thyroid hormone levels within three to six months. While awaiting the effects of the radioactive iodine, treatment with beta blockers is usually required. Antithyroid drugs, which block the production of thyroid hormone, may also be used.

In about 50% of people treated with small doses of radioactive iodine, hypothyroidism develops within the first year. A much smaller percentage (1 to 2% per year) develop hypothyroidism over the next several years. Thus hypothyroidism is a common, but acceptable, risk of treatment with radioactive iodine. However, since people treated in this way are followed closely, the diagnosis is usually made early and the replacement hormone is easy to take (one pill per day), effective, and inexpensive. A worse scenario is persistence or recurrence of hyperthyroidism, where more suffering is endured and more treatment will be required.

> Radioactive iodine must not be used during pregnancy since it can cross the placenta and could destroy the thyroid gland of the fetus.

Two different antithyroid drugs of the same class (thionamides) may be used in the treatment of Graves' hyperthyroidism. The major action is to block the synthesis of thyroid hormone. They also have a mild immune-suppressing effect; this can be beneficial in immune-mediated hyperthyroidism.

One of the antithyroid drugs, propylthiouracil (PTU) is given three times a day, whereas the other drug, methimazole (MMI), can be given once a day. We use one or the other, not both. The average doses required would be about 300 milligrams a day for PTU and 20 milligrams per day for MMI. Large doses are required for more severe disease and for larger goiters. Only low doses of PTU are used during pregnancy.

Symptoms of hyperthyroidism improve within four to six weeks of starting antithyroid drugs, but the drugs must be continued for much longer. The longer the drugs are used, the longer the remission lasts after stopping the drugs. If used for five months, only about 30% of people will remain free of symptoms, but if continued for 18 months, at least 60% will have a prolonged remission.

> The rate of recurrence of hyperthyroidism is much higher with the use of antithyroid drugs than with radioactive iodine, but the risk of hypothyroidism is much lower.

Side effects may occur with either of the antithyroid drugs. Two to five of every hundred people treated may experience itchiness of the skin, hives, rashes, or muscle and joint pain. In fewer than one in a hundred, there may be a drop in the white blood cell count. Since this drop can impair your body's ability to fight infection, the drug needs to be discontinued immediately if this side effect occurs. The white blood cell count returns to normal within one to two weeks of stopping the drug. Elderly people (over age 70) seem to be more susceptible to this particular side effect. If you are on antithyroid drugs and you develop a fever, a very bad sore throat, or a cough, you should see your physician as soon as possible to have your white blood cell count checked.

Surgical removal of most of the thyroid (subtotal thyroidectomy) is not a first line treatment for hyperthyroidism due to Graves' disease. It may be used during pregnancy, when radioactive iodine or higher doses of antithyroid drugs cannot be used. It may also be used in people with very large goiters who have failed to respond to other treatments or who cannot tolerate antithyroid drugs because of side effects.

When surgery is chosen, the frequency of non-thyroid complications is low. The possible problems include damage to the vocal cords, which may affect your voice, resulting in hoarseness, for example. There may also be (usually transient) low levels of calcium due to swelling or damage of the parathyroid glands, which lie embedded within the thyroid tissue.

Permanent hypothyroidism occurs in 25 to 75% of people within the first year of subtotal thyroidectomy. After that, it occurs at about a rate of 1% per year. A recurrence of hyperthyroidism occurs in less than 10% of people. If hypothyroidism occurs as a result of surgery, permanent replacement therapy with thyroxine will be necessary.

Treatment for Toxic Multinodular Goiter
(Multiple Toxic Nodules)

Treatment of Hyperthyroidism

Beta blockers

Radioactive iodine

Antithyroid drugs

Surgery

The treatment of choice for people with multiple toxic ("hot") nodules is radioactive iodine. Usually larger doses (20 to 30 millicuries) are given than in the treatment of Graves' disease. If the hyperthyroidism is severe, antithyroid drugs will be used for a "cooling down" period prior to treatment with the radioactive iodine. The drugs will be stopped about four days before the radioactive iodine is given. The radioactive iodine will be given as a capsule or a drink in an outpatient facility.

Unlike the situation with Graves' disease, hypothyroidism rarely occurs because is it is primarily the toxic nodules that take up the radioactive iodine. The function of the thyroid tissue around the "hot" nodules is suppressed when the nodules are functioning but can recover once the nodules have been treated.

Treatment for a Single Toxic ("Hot") Nodule

When hyperthyroidism is due to a single toxic nodule, the choices for therapy are radioactive iodine or surgical removal of the nodule. Surgery is usually employed in people under 40 and radioactive iodine in older people. Surgery is simpler in this situation because only the thyroid lobe that contains the nodule has to be removed; complications are rare. With either treatment, the risk of permanent hypothyroidism is low.

Treating Other Causes of Hyperthyroidism

TSH-secreting pituitary tumors are very rare (the rarest form of pituitary tumour) but when present cause hyperthyroidism. The treatment of hyperthyroidism due to TSH-secreting pituitary tumors involves treatment of the tumor with surgery or radiation therapy or drugs in various combinations.

CHAPTER FOUR

The Thyroid During Pregnancy and After Delivery

During Pregnancy

A mother's body undergoes many changes during pregnancy. Some of these changes, in terms of endocrinology, begin shortly after conception. For instance, levels of human chorionic gonadotropin (hCG) increase early on in pregnancy. In fact, doctors often use this change as a pregnancy test. Due to similarities in structure between hCG and TSH, hCG can stimulate the thyroid gland. Peak levels of hCG are reached near the end of the first trimester (first three months). At this time blood levels of free T4 and free T3 rise transiently and TSH levels decrease, but all levels usually remain within the normal range. In about 2% of women the levels of thyroid hormone go higher than normal and there may be symptoms of hyperthyroidism, including severe morning sickness with vomiting. The vomiting can lead to weight loss and dehydration if the condition is not treated. Often taking enough fluids and adequate rest will suffice. Occasionally beta blockers and antithyroid drugs will be needed.

The increase in hCG during pregnancy also causes an increase in the size of the thyroid, especially in iodine-deficient areas. Perhaps for this reason the ancient Egyptians used the neck circumference as a test for pregnancy. If a reed placed around a woman's neck snapped after a few weeks, she was considered to be pregnant! The "reed test" would not be successful in North America today, where there is adequate iodine and the thyroid changes very little in size during pregnancy. More iodine is required during pregnancy due to the increased needs of the mother and the fetus; however, we get enough in the diet, and supplements are not necessary.

In women with hypothyroidism who become pregnant, the dose of thyroid hormone replacement may have to be increased. With the first positive pregnancy test, your TSH should be checked and the dose of L-thyoxine increased if necessary. The increase required may be in the order of 25 to 45 %. If dosage adjustments are required, the TSH is usually measured every six to eight weeks. It is important not to take the thyroid replacement tablet at the same time as an iron or vitamin supplement as this may decrease the absorption of the hormone. Your baby's TSH level is checked in a drop of blood from a simple heel prick at the time of delivery. After delivery you can go back to your pre-pregnancy dose of thyroid hormone.

Mild hyperthyroidism is sometimes not detected in pregnancy because many of the features are similar to those that occur in normal pregnancy. These include an increase in heart rate and feeling hot. If however there is a goiter, a "stare," and a failure to gain weight, then hyperthyroidism should be suspected. Graves' disease is the usual cause and it tends to be worst in the first trimester. If not treated, there is an increased risk of miscarriage. The treatment includes adequate rest, hydration, nutrition, and antithyroid drugs, usually propylthiouracil (PTU) in low doses. Most patients will respond to therapy within one to two weeks. The dosage of PTU will be adjusted as required throughout the pregnancy. Graves' disease is less severe in the second and third trimesters. At delivery your baby's TSH level will be checked and your baby will be closely watched for signs of hyperthyroidism, such as a very rapid heart rate and hyperactivity.

If you are inadequately treated for hyperthyroidism during pregnancy, your baby will be at a greater risk for hyperthyroidism. However if you are given more PTU than your baby's thyroid can tolerate, your baby may be born with a goiter. It's a delicate balance.

Hyperthyroidism During Pregnancy

Due to hCG

Graves' disease

First Year After Delivery

Women who have had Graves' disease during pregnancy or have a past history of Graves' disease may have a relapse after delivery. If you are already on PTU, the dose may have to be increased. If you are not on antithyroid drugs and have symptoms of hyperthyroidism, your TSH should be checked.

There is also an increase in another autoimmune thyroid disease after delivery. Within one to six months of having a baby about 8% of women will experience thyroiditis (called postpartum thyroiditis). There is an initial phase of hyperthyroidism, which may last for four to six months. You may experience nervousness, irritability, a rapid heart rate, and other symptoms of hyperthyroidism. At this time, your TSH level will be low and the free T4 level increased. There will also be increased levels of antithyroid microsomal antibodies in the bloodstream. This may be followed by a hypothyroid phase of four to 12 months after delivery. The hypothyroidism is characterized by fatigue and depression and is often mistaken for postpartum depression. In the hypothyroid phase the TSH levels will be high and the free T4 levels low. There may be a transient requirement for thyroid hormone replacement for two or three months. The majority of women with postpartum thyroiditis have a return of normal thyroid function within a year of the onset of the condition. However there is a 20% chance of recurrence with subsequent pregnancies. There is also a 20% risk that the mother will develop permanent hypothyroidism due to autoimmune chronic thyroiditis.

Normal and Abnormal Thyroid Glands

Normal Thyroid

Enlarged Thyroid (Goiter)

Right
Lobe

Left
Lobe

Thyroid Nodule

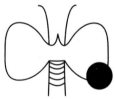

Multinodular Thyroid

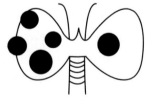

CHAPTER FIVE

Lumps and Bumps
on the Thyroid
(Thyroid Nodules)

The thyroid is a butterfly- or dumbell-shaped gland that is not usually noticeable in the neck unless it is enlarged. Lumps or bumps on the thyroid, called thyroid nodules, may be single (solitary) or there may be several of them (multinodular). The larger the nodule, the easier it is to see and to feel.

Multinodular goiters (large thyroids with many nodules) are about three times more common than single or solitary nodules.

Multinodular goiters can run in families and are more common in iodine-deficient areas, such as parts of Africa and South America. The introduction of iodized salt has eliminated iodine deficiency in most of the world, including North America. Solitary nodules are uncommon in children before puberty and are much less common in men than in women.

Nonetheless, thyroid nodules do develop, especially among certain portions of our population. For instance, thyroid nodules are more common in women and increase with age. Statistically, the lifetime risk for women of developing a nodule is between 5 and 10%. By age 75 about 9% of women have nodules that you can see or feel. By ultrasound, which is much more sensitive, 35% of these women have thyroid nodules!

Most of these nodules are found by chance and are no reason for concern.

People tend to be more aware of a multinodular goiter than a solitary nodule. Nodules may be noted during a doctor's examination or by someone sitting across from you, or by yourself when looking in a mirror. In fact, you can do a personal neck check in the following manner:

1. Expose your neck (no high collars or turtlenecks).
2. Have a glass of water handy.
3. Look in a mirror and focus on your neck, in the region above your collarbone and below your voice box or Adam's apple. (The thyroid is a little higher up in a woman's neck than in a man's neck.) The Adam's apple is the bump that you can see in most people; it is normal.
4. Take a drink of water and as you swallow look for the thyroid gland, which moves up as you swallow. Both lobes of the thyroid (one on either side of the windpipe) and the isthmus (or bridge that stretches across the windpipe) will move with swallowing.
5. If you see any lumps, bumps, or bulges of the thyroid, have your doctor check it out. But don't panic; you are very unlikely to discover anything serious.

Self-examination of the Thyroid

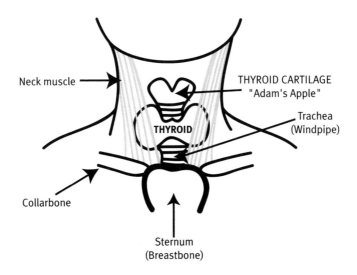

The majority of people with multinodular goiters have no symptoms. Hypothyroidism is rarely seen with this condition. More commonly, some of the nodules will be "autonomous," that is, they will make and release thyroid hormone without responding to the normal hierarchy of hypothalamic–pituitary–thyroid regulation. The TSH may be low, with normal thyroid hormone levels. However, over the years, as the nodules grow and produce more thyroid hormone, there is a risk of hyperthyroidism due to the "toxic" or "hot" nodules.

If a multinodular goiter is extremely large, you may have problems with swallowing, breathing, or with your voice. Report these things to your doctor. The increase in neck size may also make it difficult to button up a collar!

Most people with solitary nodules have no symptoms and are totally unaware that they have the nodule. Thyroid function in the rest of the gland is usually normal. Rarely the nodule will be a "toxic" or "hot" nodule and cause hyperthyroidism.

If solitary nodules are more than four centimetres in size, they are a little more conspicuous. They will also be more likely to cause neck symptoms and more likely to be malignant (cancer-containing). If there is hoarseness and a nodule appears to be growing rapidly, the risk of cancer is greater.

Laboratory Testing

Lab tests for Thyroid Nodules

TSH

Fine needle aspiration biopsy

Other

As for other thyroid conditions, the initial screening test for thyroid nodules is measurement of TSH. If the TSH is low, then levels of free T4 and free T3 will be done to check for hyperthyroidism. If the TSH is high, levels of free T4 and thyroid antibodies will be done to check for hypothyroidism and a possible autoimmune cause for the hypothyroidism.

Most people with solitary nodules will have a normal

TSH. Your doctor may then proceed to do a fine needle aspiration biopsy of the nodule. This is done to determine whether the nodule is benign or malignant.

The fine needle aspiration biopsy may be done in the doctor's office or by a radiologist; a thyroid ultrasound may be done at the same time to be sure the needle is in the nodule. The neck is first cleaned with an antiseptic solution. A small needle (smaller than the one used for drawing blood), which is attached to a plastic syringe, is inserted into the nodule. Suction is applied with the syringe at various angles while the needle is in the nodule. There may be a sensation of pressure but the procedure is usually only mildly painful. The needle is withdrawn and the material that has been collected is placed on a glass microscope slide. A pathologist examines the slides, gives a description of the thyroid cells (the science of cytology), and interprets the material as benign, suspicious, or malignant. There is about a 5% chance that a solitary nodule will be malignant (cancer); in other words, there is a 95% chance that it will be benign (not cancer).

Traditionally, thyroid scans have been done with either radioiodine or technetium to determine whether thyroid nodules are nonfunctioning ("cold") nodules. "Hot" (functioning) nodules are typically benign. In the past, a fine needle aspiration would have been done on a "cold" nodule, but not a "hot" nodule. These days, if the TSH is normal, many endocrinologists will skip the thyroid scan and go immediately to the fine needle aspiration biopsy, which is reasonably accurate with very little risk.

Ultrasound can be very useful in determining whether a solitary nodule is indeed solitary or whether there are other nodules that are present but are not large enough to be felt. We can usually feel nodules that are one centimetre or greater in size. The presence of multiple nodules makes malignancy (cancer) much less likely.

Ultrasound can also be used to determine whether the nodule is cystic (fluid-filled; usually benign) or solid (occasionally malignant). It also gives a more accurate measure of the size of the nodule(s) and can be used in monitoring the growth of the nodule over time, if it is not to be removed.

In nodules that are larger than three centimetres, there is a greater risk of abnormalities, both at the time they are found and in the future. In people with solitary nodules larger than three centimetres there will be a greater risk of cancer. In people with multinodular goiters who have a nodule bigger than three centimetres, there is a somewhat greater risk that the nodule will become overactive with time and cause hyperthyroidism.

Typically, nodules less than one centimetre in size are not biopsied because of the low risk of finding anything worrisome.

Fine needle aspiration biopsy is recommended for solitary nodules that are one centimetre in diameter or longer.

Treatment

If a fine needle aspiration is done and the pathologist's report states that the cytology (appearance of the cells) is benign, the treatment options include simple observation over time or observation during a time-limited (e.g., 6 to 12 months) trial of L-thyroxine to see whether the nodule can be decreased in size.

Smaller nodules are easier to suppress. Enough L-thyroxine is added to suppress your own TSH level to the lower limits of normal or just below normal. Any changes in the size of the nodule are assessed by palpation (examination with fingers) and ultrasound.

If the nodule increases in size while on L-thyroxine, it needs to be evaluated further. If the nodule decreases in size, then the choice may be made to continue the L-thyroxine therapy. If there is no change in the nodule after 6 or 12 months of L-thyroxine, then the choice may be made to stop this type of therapy.

Sometimes the pathologist's report states that the cytology is suspicious for cancer or is malignant. If this should occur, then thyroid surgery will be required for a final diagnosis and for treatment. During surgery, if the "suspicious" nodule is benign, then the half of the thyroid that contains the nodule is removed. If it is cancerous, then more extensive surgery will be done.

Assuming that the nodule turns out to be benign, you may be discharged from hospital the same day or within a day or two. Consideration will be given to adding L-thyroxine on a daily basis in an attempt to prevent other thyroid nodules from developing on the other side (the other lobe of thyroid).

The scar from simple thyroid surgery is usually a fine line at the base of the neck (often called a "necklace" or "collar" scar), and if desired can be covered with a necklace once it has healed.

CHAPTER SIX

Thyroid Cancer and
Life After Thyroid Cancer

Clinical Facts

Thyroid cancer is rare, making up only about 1% of all kinds of cancer. Thyroid cancer usually appears as a thyroid nodule. Ordinarily, there are no symptoms of over- or underactivity of the thyroid gland. The treatment of thyroid cancer usually involves surgery and radioactive iodine. The response to treatment is excellent for the majority of people who have been found to have thyroid cancer.

Solitary thyroid nodules have a 5 to 10% risk of being malignant (cancerous). Nodules in a multinodular goiter have only about a 1% risk of having cancer. Thyroid cancer is even more rare in people who have had a previous history of Hashimoto's thyroiditis or Graves' disease.

There are certain factors that appear to predispose people to the development of thyroid cancer. Most thyroid diseases, including thyroid cancer, are more common in women. However, solitary thyroid nodules in men or in children under 14 have a much greater risk of cancer than do solitary nodules in women. Almost half of the thyroid nodules found in children are malignant. The thyroid cancers found in people over the age of 50 tend to be more aggressive.

Thyroid cancer is more likely to be found in hard, irregular, solitary nodules, especially if they seem to be "fixed" or stuck down to other tissues in the neck. If there are enlarged lymph nodes in the neck, this also increases the suspicion for malignancy. If the nodule appears to be growing and causing symptoms such as trouble swallowing or trouble breathing, the risk of cancer is higher.

Exposure to external radiation increases the risk of thyroid cancer. The radiation may have been for treatment of benign or malignant disease in the region of the head/neck/chest or from exposure to radioactive fallout as with the atomic bomb in Japan or nuclear accidents such as at Chernobyl, Russia. It has been estimated that about 14% of people who have had radiation to the neck will develop thyroid cancer. There is also an increase in the incidence of benign thyroid nodules after radiation to the neck.

However, internal radiation from radioactive iodine in the doses that are used to treat Graves' disease does not appear to increase the risk of thyroid cancer.

Rarely, genetic factors can increase the risk of thyroid cancer in families; medullary cancer of the thyroid is a particular example.

Laboratory Testing

A screening TSH is done in patients suspected of having thyroid cancer but this is usually normal. If medullary carcinoma of the thyroid is suspected, measurements of the hormone calcitonin will be done. Genetic testing for this rare condition is suggested when there is a strong family history of medullary cancer of the thyroid. Such genetic testing is done primarily in research laboratories.

**Thyroid Cancer
Types and Growth Rates**

Papillary—slow

Follicular—slow

Medullary—moderate;
metastases common

Anaplastic—rapid;
metastases common

Various types of imaging such as thyroid scanning with radioactive iodine or technetium, ultrasound, computerized tomography (CT scanning), or even magnetic resonance imaging (MRI) may be done to evaluate a neck lump.

Fine needle aspiration biopsy of the nodule is usually the next step to help make the diagnosis. Spread of malignant cells along the needle tract has not been shown to be a problem with this technique. If the biopsy specimen is suspicious for malignancy or shows cancer cells, thyroid surgery will be required.

Treatment

If the thyroid nodule is malignant, the extent of the surgical treatment and other treatments will depend on the type of cancer found.

The cancers that arise from the follicular cells of the thyroid are papillary carcinoma, follicular carcinoma, and anaplastic carcinoma. Cancers that arise from the parafollicular cells (C-cells) of the thyroid are called medullary carcinoma.

Papillary and follicular cancers have a slow rate of growth, medullary cancers a moderate rate, and anaplastic cancers a very rapid rate of growth.

Papillary carcinoma is by far the most commonly diagnosed thyroid cancer, making up almost 75% of cases. It is three times more common in women than in men. The tumor is slow growing. It may spread to lymph nodes in the neck, but spread to bones and lungs is much less common. It is, however, not unusual for the cancer to have spread within the thyroid gland, to the opposite lobe, for example.

Overall, the prognosis for people with thyroid cancer is good. Less than 10% of people with papillary carcinoma die of the disease. Only about 25% have a recurrence of the cancer after treatment, and most of the recurrences can be successfully treated.

If the size of the papillary cancer found at surgery is

less than one centimetre, the affected thyroid lobe and the isthmus will be removed. For tumors that are larger than this, a subtotal or near-total thyroidectomy will be done.

If there is spread of the cancer (metastases) to lymph glands (nodes) in the neck, the nodes will be removed in what is called a modified neck dissection. The more extensive the surgery, the greater the risk for damage to the parathyroid glands (embedded in the thyroid) and to the recurrent laryngeal nerve, which is the nerve to the voice box. If the parathyroid glands are damaged or removed, there is a risk for low calcium levels in the blood. Calcium and Vitamin D supplements may be needed to restore calcium levels to normal. If the laryngeal nerve is damaged there may be hoarseness of your voice. This may be permanent.

For papillary cancers that are 1.5 centimetres or larger, radioactive iodine (I131) is given after surgery (usually four to six weeks later) to ablate (wipe out) any remaining thyroid tissue. The dose of radioactive iodine is variable, but about 100 millicuries (mC) is used if there is no spread of the tumor, 150 mC if there are neck nodes, and 200 mC if there is spread outside the neck.

In preparation for the radioactive iodine, you will likely be admitted to a private room in a hospital. After you swallow the radioactive iodine capsule or liquid, you will have to remain in your room until discharge, usually 48 hours later. During the stay, a nuclear medicine technologist will visit you regularly to measure the level of radiation in your body. You can read, watch TV, talk on the phone, etc.; meals are brought in. You will be encouraged to drink 8 to 12 glasses of fluid each day. This increases urination and speeds up excretion (washing out) of any radioactive iodine that has not been picked up by thyroid tissue. You can suck on sour candies to increase saliva and prevent a dry mouth. Medication can be given to you for nausea but is usually not necessary.

After discharge following radioactive iodine treatment, it is suggested that you use separate disposable eating utensils for about four days. It is also a good idea to "keep at arm's length" from others and to sleep alone for the first week. Also, minimize time spent with children and pregnant women in the first week following treatment. The reason for these suggestions is that your body is slightly radioactive for a few days.

A whole body scan is done one week after the therapeutic dose of I131 is administered to see where the iodine was picked up as an indication of tumor spread. Thyroid hormone is then started, both to replace the missing thyroid and to provide enough hormone to suppress the TSH level below normal. There is evidence to show that this so-called suppressive therapy with thyroid hormone will decrease the recurrence/reappearance of the cancer. External radiation therapy may be used in people who have been treated surgically and with radioactive iodine but are no longer responding to radioactive iodine.

Follicular cancer, which makes up about 15% of thyroid cancers, is more aggressive than papillary cancer and can spread through the blood stream to cause distant metastases to bone, liver or brain. Older people, and those whose tumors have spread outside the thyroid gland, tend to do more poorly. But this is a generalization, and may not apply to you.

The surgery for follicular cancer usually involves a near-total or total thyroidectomy (removal of the thyroid). As with papillary carcinoma, radioactive iodine is used after surgery to ablate (destroy) any remaining thyroid tissue. Higher doses are used to treat metastases if the metastases can pick up or concentrate iodine. External radiotherapy may be used if the tumor fails to concentrate iodine. Suppressive doses of thyroid hormone (L-thyroxine) are used in an attempt to prevent recurrence of the cancer.

Anaplastic cancer, a very aggressive form of thyroid cancer, makes up 5% or less of thyroid cancers and tends to occur in people over the age of 50. Over the age of 80, about 50% of newly diagnosed thyroid cancers will be anaplastic.

By the time anaplastic cancer is discovered, it has usually spread extensively. Surgery may be required to prevent the tumor from obstructing your airway. When complete tumor removal is not possible, local "debulking" surgery may be done to remove as much of the tumor as possible, so that you can breathe and swallow.

External radiation (4000 to 5000 rads) is given to the neck to attempt tumor shrinkage. Chemotherapy with doxorubicin or bleomycin or other drugs may also be tried. Unfortunately, results are poor and most patients die within about seven months from the time of diagnosis of anaplastic thyroid cancer.

Thyroid lymphoma makes up about 1% of thyroid cancers. It may occur more frequently in people with a past history of Hashimoto's thyroiditis. If the lymphoma is confined to the thyroid, total thyroidectomy can be done. More often, however, the disease has spread and radiation therapy or chemotherapy are used for treatment of the lymphoma. Thyroid hormone can be easily replaced but the overall outcome will depend on how well the lymphoma responds to the cancer treatments.

Medullary carcinoma of the thyroid accounts for about 5 to 10% of thyroid cancer. Males and females of all ages can be affected. About 20% of the cases are familial (hereditary) and may be associated with other endocrine tumors. Medullary cancer commonly metastasizes (spreads) to neck nodes and to distant sites (lung, bones, and liver). The tumor produces large amounts of the hormone calcitonin, which can be measured in the blood.

The initial treatment for medullary carcinoma of the thyroid is a near-total thyroidectomy with removal of lymph nodes in the neck. These tumors do not usually pick up iodine, so radioactive iodine is not a treatment option. The role of external radiation therapy is controversial. In other words, the only effective therapy we have at present is surgery.

Follow-up

Immediate follow-up after surgical treatment for thyroid cancer involves monitoring the neck incision to make sure there is no local obstruction to breathing and checking the blood calcium levels. Within 24 to 48 hours after a total or near-total thyroidectomy, there may be a drop in the calcium level due to unintentional injury or removal of the parathyroid glands. The parathyroid glands consist of four small spherical glands that are embedded in the four corners (top and bottom of both lobes) of the thyroid gland. The parathyroids secrete a hormone called parathyroid hormone (PTH), which is involved in the regulation of calcium. Too much PTH causes high blood levels of calcium and too little PTH results in low levels of calcium. Injury of the parathyroids may result in a transient hypoparathyroidism (underactivity of the parathyroid glands), while complete removal of all four glands would result in permanent hypoparathyroidism.

The risk of hypoparathyroidism is clearly linked to the extent of the surgery. When thyroid cancer is more widespread in the neck and more aggressive surgery is required for removal, there will be a greater risk. The symptoms of a mild decrease in calcium include tingling around the mouth and in the hands and feet. This responds to extra calcium given by mouth. With larger drops in calcium there may be muscle spasms, especially in the hands. In these cases, the calcium is replaced through an intravenous line as well as by mouth until the symptoms have gone. In transient hypoparathyroidism the calcium supplement will be given for only a short period of time, but in permanent hypoparathyroidism it will be required for life. Vitamin D by mouth is also added to help increase the absorption of the calcium and maintain the calcium levels in the normal range.

> People who have been treated for thyroid cancer require life-long monitoring since recurrences can occur decades after the initial treatment.

Most patients with papillary or follicular cancer are treated with surgery followed by radioactive iodine ablation (destruction) and thyroid hormone suppression therapy. TSH levels will be monitored to make sure they are suppressed. The dose of L-thyroxine will be adjusted to achieve suppression of TSH. Thyroglobulin (Tg) is measured as a "tumor marker." If there has been complete ablation of thyroid tissue, there should be no functioning thyroid tissue and the level of thyroglobulin should be undetectable. However, in as many as 25% of people with thyroid cancer, there may be interference with the Tg assay by Tg antibodies (Tgab). Tgab can cause either an under- or overestimation of the Tg level. Newer and more accurate methods of measuring thyroglobulin production are under investigation.

Rather than using a normal range, your Tg levels are monitored for changes. If there is a significant increase in the Tg level, patients are usually taken off their thyroid hormone, allowed to become transiently hypothyroid, reflected by an elevation in TSH. A radioiodine whole body scan is then done to look for tumor recurrence. In future, the more ready availability of recombinant human thyroid-stimulating hormone (rhTSH) may speed up this process by allowing patients to stay on thyroid hormone. This would also avoid the uncomfortable symptoms of hypothyroidism that go along with our current approach.

If there is evidence of recurrent thyroid cancer that picks up iodine, then further radioactive iodine treatments can be given. If there is no iodine uptake, external radiation can be considered.

People who have been treated for medullary carcinoma of the thyroid are assessed on a regular basis with physical examinations and measurement of calcitonin levels. If the calcitonin levels begin to rise, further investigation is required. Computerized tomography (CT), or magnetic resonance imaging (MRI) may be employed in an attempt to determine the location of a tumor recurrence. The five year survival rate for medullary carcinoma of thyroid is about 80%.

The five year survival rate for papillary and follicular carcinoma is about 95%. Patients treated for papillary or follicular cancer have a 30-year survival rate of about 75% when a combination of surgery, radioactive iodine, and thyroid hormone suppression therapy is used. This may improve even further as we develop more sensitive assays for detecting residual or recurrent cancer. Younger people with smaller tumors tend to do better than people over 60 or people with larger tumors at the time of diagnosis.

Case History A

A 48-year-old woman went to see her family doctor because of severe cold symptoms, including a cough and sore throat. While checking the neck for swollen and tender lymph nodes, as one may find with respiratory infections, her doctor found a thyroid nodule. She didn't have any symptoms of hyperthyroidism or hypothyroidism and her TSH level was normal. She was referred to an endocrinologist who did a biopsy of the cherry-sized thyroid nodule. The pathology report suggested that it was papillary carcinoma of the thyroid. She was then referred to a surgeon who saw her in consultation and made plans for a near-total thyroidectomy. The surgery went smoothly and she was discharged the morning of the third day after surgery. The surgical pathology report confirmed the diagnosis of a papillary cancer 2.5 cm (1 in.) in size and did not reveal any spread elsewhere in the thyroid or in lymph nodes in the neck.

She then went back to her endocrinologist who booked a room in the hospital for a two-day admission about six weeks later. During the wait for her hospitalization she was feeling more tired than usual and gained five pounds. The TSH level done a few days before her admission to hospital was very elevated. The endocrinologist was happy with this result as it meant that if there were any remaining thyroid cells, they would very avidly pick up the radioactive iodine that would be given as further treatment for the cancer.

At the hospital, she was asked to swallow the radioactive iodine (I131) capsule and then instructed to drink 8 to 12 glasses of water a day and to stay in her own room. There was an adjoining bathroom that she made good use of considering the amount of water she was drinking. Her meals were brought to her and she enjoyed reading a book and watching TV. Her nurses and doctors popped in and out but nobody stayed long because of the radioactivity. However the radioactive counts, which were frequently monitored, went steadily down and she was discharged home within 48 hours of entering the hospital.

The woman returned as an out-patient one week after the I131 had been given to have a whole body scan. Fortunately, the scan did not show any spread of the thyroid cancer. She was started on levothyroxine as a replacement thyroid hormone, since she no longer had a thyroid gland. The dose was adjusted until her TSH level was suppressed just below the normal range and her free T4 level was in the normal range. Suppression of TSH helps to suppress the growth of any tumor cells that may be left behind.

Six months after the surgery her endocrinologist could not feel any recurrence of the cancer in the neck. The thyroglobulin level, which is used as a tumor marker, was undetectable. This is what you would expect after a thyroidectomy when there is no normal or abnormal (cancerous) thyroid tissue left. One year after the surgery the incision site on her neck is just a fine line. She feels "back to normal."

Case History B

A 63-year-old woman had been followed by an endocrinologist for many years. She had a multinodular goiter with a dominant or much larger nodule on one side. Her endocrinologist had just retired so she changed to a new one, who requested a thyroid ultrasound to be compared with the previous ones. At the same time as the ultrasound was done, a needle biopsy was taken from the dominant nodule, which appeared to have enlarged since the last ultrasound. The cytology report suggested papillary cancer and she was referred for surgical removal of the thyroid gland.

After the operation, her calcium levels dropped and the dosages of her calcium and vitamin D supplements had to be increased. The final pathology report revealed a 3.5 cm papillary cancer without any spread elsewhere in the neck.

She subsequently was treated with radioactive iodine and replaced with enough thyroxine to suppress her TSH. She continues to do well, although it took some time to normalize her calcium level, which was finally accomplished with the addition of a vitamin D preparation called calcitriol (Rocaltrol).

The Future

While future research and medical developments in treating thyroid disease are hard to predict, here is a list of six improvements we should be able to expect in the years ahead.

1. Adequate iodine to prevent iodine-deficiency goiter in all parts of the world.
2. Better methods of detecting thyroid cancer with the use of biological and immunological markers.
3. More "patient-friendly" ways of treating thyroid cancer, both surgically and medically. This will include being able to eliminate the prolonged hypothyroid phase before treatment with radioactive iodine.
4. Fine tuning of thyroid hormone replacement therapy, particularly in people who are depressed or continue to have symptoms of hypothyroidism with the usual replacement therapy.
5. A better understanding of autoimmune thyroid disease so that we can prevent it or cure it rather than just treat it. This could eliminate the most common thyroid problems.

6. An appreciation of the beauty and complexity of thyroid hormone action with a steady growth of knowledge and useful applications of that knowledge.

Glossary of Terms

Acute

Starting quickly. Something that is acute does not have to be severe; it can be mild, moderate, or severe.

Anaplastic Thyroid Carcinoma

A very rare and aggressive form of thyroid cancer.

Antibodies

Substances produced by the immune system in response to something that it considers foreign to the body. Autoantibodies are antibodies produced against our own tissues. This is abnormal and is called autoimmune disease.

Aspirate

To draw fluid out by suction, usually through a needle attached to a syringe.

Autoimmune Disease

A disease associated with antibodies to our own tissue/organs. Endocrine examples would include Graves' disease, Hashimoto's thyroiditis, and Type 1 (early onset) diabetes. A non-endocrine example would be lupus.

Benign

Not malignant (not cancer).

Beta Blocker Drugs

Drugs that block the actions of epinephrine (adrenaline) and norepinephrine (noradrenaline), thereby reducing the heart and pulse rate, blood pressure, tremors, and anxiety.

Biopsy

Removal of a piece of tissue for microscopic examination and diagnosis.

C Cells

Cells of the thyroid gland that produce a hormone called calcitonin. The C cells are also called parafollicular cells.

Calcitonin

A hormone produced by the thyroid gland. It is involved in the regulation of calcium in the body. Calcitonin is produced in excess by medullary carcinoma of the thyroid.

Capsule   An enclosing membrane.

Chronic   Long lasting.

Clavicle   Collarbone.

Colloid   A thick and viscous substance in the
                        center of the thyroid follicular cells.
                        Thyroid hormone is stored there.

Computerized   A form of x-ray technology in which
Tomography (CT)   images are taken in slices throughout
                        the organ or body. It may also be
                        called a CAT scan (computerized
                        axial tomography).

Congenital   Existing at birth.

Cretin   Person with severe hypothyroidism,
                        present at the time of birth, resulting
                        in mental and other defects.

Cyst   A sac containing liquid matter,
                        surrounded by a capsule.

Deficiency   Lack or shortage of.

Deiodination   Removal of iodine from a compound.

Drugs   In this book we are referring to
                        medications or medical substances.

Dysfunction	Abnormal function.
Endocrine Glands	Glands that secrete hormones and other substances into the blood stream.
Endocrinologist	A doctor who specializes in the treatment of endocrine (hormonal) conditions.
Epinephrine	Also called adrenaline. It is a hormone secreted by the adrenal gland.
Euthyroid: ***"Clinically*** ***Euthyroid"***	The patient has no signs or symptoms of an over- or under-active thyroid.
"Biochemically ***Euthyroid"***	The state of normal thyroid hormone levels, which may be produced naturally or be provided with replacement medications.
Feedback ***Mechanism***	A mechanism that is regulated by its own products. Negative feedback involves suppression, and positive feedback, stimulation.
Follicular ***Carcinoma***	A type of thyroid cancer which can spread through the bloodstream.

Follicules	Also called follicles. In this book, they refer to the cells of the thyroid gland that produce thyroid hormone.
Goiter	An enlargement of the thyroid gland.
Graves' Disease	An autoimmune disorder in which thyroid-stimulating antibodies increase the growth of the thyroid gland and the production of thyroid hormone. It is the most common cause of hyperthyroidism.
Hashimoto's Disease	An autoimmune disease in which antibodies are associated with destruction of the thyroid gland and decreased production of thyroid hormone. It is the most common cause of hypothyroidism.
Hormones	Substances produced by the endocrine glands and released into the blood stream. They may have local effects or far distant and far ranging effects in the body. You can think of hormones as chemical messengers.

Hyperthyroidism A disease resulting from an overactive thyroid gland with excess secretion of thyroid hormone. Common symptoms include nervous-ness, anxiety, weight loss, feeling hot, and a rapid heart rate pulse. (Hyper is a prefix meaning "over.")

Hypothalamus A part of the brain that secretes thyrotropin releasing hormone (TRH), which stimulates another part of the brain (the pituitary gland), located just beneath it, to produce thyroid-stimulating hormone (TSH).

Hypothyroidism A disease resulting from an underactive thyroid gland with inadequate production of thyroid hormone. Common symptoms include fatigue, weight gain, sensitivity to the cold, constipation, and dry skin. ("Hypo" is a prefix meaning "under".)

Iodine A chemical that is absorbed from the diet and water which the thyroid gland uses to help make thyroid hormone. Small amounts of iodine are essential for the production of thyroid hormone.

Isthmus   A connection between two larger
                         areas. The isthmus of the thyroid
                         connects the right and left halves
                         (lobes).

L-thyroxine   A synthetic thyroid hormone that is
                         the same as the thyroxine normally
                         produced by the thyroid gland. It is
                         used as replacement therapy for
                         hypothyroidism and to suppress the
                         growth of benign thyroid nodules
                         and malignant thyroid tissue.

Larynx   Part of the throat in which the vocal
                         cords are located; voice box.

Lobe   Part of an organ. The thyroid gland
                         has two similar lobes, on each side of
                         the windpipe. The lobes of the
                         thyroid are connected by a thin band
                         of tissue called the isthmus.

Lymphadenopathy   Enlargement of one or more lymph
                         nodes.

Lymphatic System   A system of tubes and kidney-bean-
                         shaped glands throughout the body,
                         which make up part of the immune
                         system of the body.

Lymphoma	A type of cancer affecting the tissues of the lymphatic system, mainly the lymph glands (nodes).
Magnetic Resonance Imaging (MRI)	(Also known as MR) Creating images of the body by a combination of a magnetic field and radiofrequency signals. Unlike x-rays, there is no radiation exposure.
Malignant	Cancerous.
Medullary Carcinoma of the Thyroid	A rare type of thyroid cancer affecting the parafollicular or C cells, which make the hormone calcitonin.
Menstruation	Monthly loss of blood from the uterus, from puberty to menopause; also called "periods."
Metabolism	The chemical processes by which we produce energy.
Myxedema	An old term for hypothyroidism or underactive thyroid; also used to describe an abnormal skin lesion that may be seen on the legs or feet of people with Graves' hyperthyroidism (e.g., pretibial myxedema).

Norepinephrine	Also called noradrenaline. It is a hormone produced in the adrenal glands and in the sympathetic nervous system.
Normalize	To make normal; to restore to the usual state or level.
Papillary Carcinoma	The most common type of thyroid cancer. It can spread through the lymphatic system, to lymph nodes in the neck, for example.
Parathyroid Glands	Four small glands in the region of the thyroid gland in the neck. They produce a hormone called parathyroid hormone.
Parathyroid Hormone	A hormone produced by the parathyroid glands. It is involved in the regulation of calcium levels in the body. Excess may produce high blood calcium levels (hypercalcemia), and deficiency may produce low blood calcium levels (hypocalcemia).

Pituitary Gland   A small gland, called the "master gland," which is actually part of the brain. It sits in a little bony cup (the sella), which is located just above the back of the nose. It produces many hormones, including thyroid stimulating hormone (TSH), which stimulates the thyroid gland to produce thyroid hormone.

Plasma   The part of the blood without the blood cells.

Postpartum   After delivery of a baby.

Precursor Hormones   The larger "prohormones" that give rise to the circulating active hormones.

Radio-immunoassay Technique   A technique that uses small amounts of radioactivity to trace or measure small amounts of substances in the blood or tissues.

Radioiodine   Radioactive iodine. When it is absorbed by the thyroid gland, electromagnetic waves are produced, which cause ejection of electrons (ionizing radiation). It is used in testing thyroid function and in treating some thyroid diseases.

Radiotherapy	Treatment of disease by x-rays or other forms of radiation.
Replacement Therapy	Therapy that replaces or substitutes for a natural substance.
Scan	To obtain an image (e.g., of a part of the body).
Sternum	Central bone in the chest; breastbone.
Subacute	Coming quickly, but not as quickly as "acute."
Subtotal Thyroidectomy	Removal of more than 75 percent of the thyroid gland.
T3, free T3	Short forms for tri-iodothyronine and free tri-iodothyronine, which is tri-iodothyronine that is not bound to proteins and is thus free to be biologically active.
T4, free T4	Short forms for thyroxine and free thyroxine, which is thyroxine that is not bound to proteins and is thus free to be biologically active. Thyroxine is the major hormone produced by the thyroid gland.

Technetium   A radioactive metallic element used
in certain types of scans.

Thyroglobulin   The large protein-carbohydrate
(Tg)   molecule or compound produced by
functioning thyroid tissue and stored
in colloid within the thyroid gland. It
is the precursor of the thyroid
hormones.

Thyroid Gland   A butterfly- or dumbbell-shaped
gland that is located in the neck. It
sits on top of the windpipe between
the voice box and the collarbone. It
produces thyroid hormones.

Thyroid   The hormones thyroxine (T4) and
Hormones   tri-iodothyronine (T3), which are
produced by the thyroid gland. They
modify the body's rate of metabolism.
An excess speeds up the rate and
deficiencies slow the rate.

Thyroid Nodules   Abnormal lumps or bumps that may
be felt on the thyroid gland. They
may be cystic (fluid-filled) or solid.
The cysts and multiples of the solids
are usually benign in nature. Single or
solitary growths will be malignant
(containing cancer) about 5 to 10% of
the time.

Thyroiditis

A subacute or chronic disorder of the thyroid gland. The subacute forms may be inflammatory in origin or due to autoimmune disease and cause hyperthyroidism followed by hypothyroidism and then a return to normal thyroid function over months.

Tissue

Collections of cells (small units of living matter).

Trachea

Windpipe.

Transient

Passing; of short duration.

TRH

Short form for thyrotropin releasing hormone. It is produced by the hypothalamus.

Trimester

A three-month period of time. The human pregnancy, which lasts nine months, is divided into three trimesters, the first, second, and third.

TSH

Short form for thyroid stimulating hormone. It is produced by the pituitary.

Tumor

An abnormal growth of tissue. However, technically, it simply means "a lump."

Ultrasound	The use of ultrasonic waves to study an organ. Ultrasonic waves are sound waves above the range of normal hearing.
Variant	A different form.
Viruses	Extremely small organisms that can replicate (produce copies of themselves) within the cells of a host body such as the human body. They may cause a wide range of diseases.

Drugs Commonly Used
in Thyroid Disorders

Reason for Use	Generic Name	Trade Name(s)
Hypothyroidism	levothroxine (l-thyroxine)	Synthroid Eltroxin Levothroid Levoxyl Levotec
	tri-iodothyronine	Cytomel
Hyperthyroidism	propylthiouracil (PTU)	Propyl-Thyracil
	methimazole (MMI)	Tapazole
	propranolol	Inderal
		Inderal-LA Apo-Propranolol Nu-Propranolol
	I131 (radioactive iodine)	I131
Thyroid cancer	I131	I131

Resources

Thyroid Foundation of Canada

Originally founded in Kingston, Ontario; now there are chapters across Canada.

Local branches should be in the telephone book.

Kingston phone number:	1-800-267-8822
	or (613) 634-3426
Fax number:	(613) 632-3483
Website:	www.io.org/~thyroid/Canada.html
email:	thyroid@io.org

Thyroid Foundation of America, Inc.

Headquarters in Boston, Massachusetts, with chapters across the United States.

Boston phone number:	1-800-832-8321
	or (617) 726-8500
Fax number:	(617) 726-4136
Website:	www.tsh.org
email:	tfa@clark.net

Thyroid Society for Education and Research
Based in Houston, Texas.

Phone number:	1-800-THYROID
	(1-800-849-7643)
	or (713) 799-9909
Fax number:	(713) 779-9919
Website:	www.the-thyroid-society.org

American Association of Clinical Endocrinologists
Headquarters in Jacksonville, Florida.

Phone number:	(904) 353-7878
Fax number:	(904) 353-8185
Website:	www.aace.com

American Thyroid Association Inc.
Headquarters in Bronx, New York.

Phone number:	(718) 882-6047
FAX number:	(718) 882-6085
Website:	www.thyroid.org
email:	info@thyroid.org

The Endocrine Society
Headquarters in Bethesda, Maryland.

Phone number:	(301) 941-0200
Fax number:	(301) 941-0259
	or 1-888-ENDOFAX
Website:	www.endo-society.org

Thyroid Foundation International

Headquarters in Kingston, Ontario.

    Phone number: (613) 544-8364

    Fax number: (613) 544-9731

    Website: www.thyroid-fed.org/home.html

    email: tfi@kos.net

Endocrinologist-operated Website

Dr. Daniel Drucker, thyroid specialist at the Toronto Hospital (University of Toronto):

    Website: www.mythyroid.com

Pharmaceutical-operated Website

Knoll Pharmaceutical Company: Synthroid

    Website: www.yourthyroid.com

Other sources that will be in the telephone book:

Canadian Cancer Society

American Cancer Society

Index

For over fifty years, Coles Notes have been helping
students get through high school and university.
New Coles Notes will help get you through the rest of life.

Look for these NEW COLES NOTES!

BUSINESS
- Effective Business Presentations
- Accounting for Small Business
- Write Effective Business Letters
- Write a Great Résumé
- Do A Great Job Interview
- Start Your Own Small Business
- Get Ahead at Work

PERSONAL FINANCE
- Basic Investing
- Investing in Stocks
- Investing in Mutual Funds
- Buying and Selling Your Home
- Plan Your Estate
- Develop a Personal Financial Plan

LIFESTYLE
- Wine
- Bartending
- Beer
- Wedding
- Opera
- Casino Gambling
- Better Bridge
- Better Chess
- Better Golf
- Better Tennis
- Public Speaking
- Speed Reading
- Cooking 101
- Scholarships and Bursaries
- Cats and Cat Care
- Dogs and Dog Care
- Writing to Get Published

PARENTING
- Your Child: The First Year
- Your Child: The Terrific Twos
- Your Child: Ages Three and Four
- Your Child: Age Five to Eight
- Your Child: Age Nine to Twelve
- Your Child: The Teenage Years
- Raising A Reader
- Helping Your Child in Math

SPORTS FOR KIDS
- Basketball for Kids
- Baseball for Kids
- Soccer for Kids
- Gymnastics for Kids
- Martial Arts for Kids

PHRASE BOOKS
- French
- Spanish
- Italian
- German
- Russian
- Japanese
- Greek

GARDENING
- Indoor Gardening
- Perennial Gardening
- Herb Gardening
- Organic Gardening

MEDICAL SERIES
- Prostate Cancer
- Breast Cancer
- Thyroid Problems

**Coles Notes and New Coles Notes are available at the following stores:
Chapters • Coles • World's Biggest Bookstore**